KEFıʀ

12 Fast And Easy Kefir Diet Recipes For Rapid Weight Loss, Avoiding Mistakes & Feeling Amazing

Contents

The trademarks that are used are without any consent, and the publication of the trademark is without permission or backing by the trademark owner. All trademarks and brands within this book are for clarifying purposes only and are the owned by the owners themselves, not affiliated with this document.

Introduction

I want to thank you and congratulate You for purchasing the book, *"Kefir: 12 Fast and Easy Kefir Diet Recipes for Weight Loss, Avoid Mistakes & Feel Amazing"*.

This book contains simple steps on how to make Kefir at home and lose weight using fast & easy 12 Kefir diet recipes. By reading this book you will discover:

- Connection between probiotics and obesity
- Probiotics impact to weight loss
- Amazing benefits of Kefir
- Top strategies of losing weight with Kefir for obese people
- Best recipes for a healthy intestinal flora
- Some great tips for losing weight & avoiding mistakes

We all already know that probiotics are bacteria that are naturally found in the intestine of every human being and make the intestinal microflora, which protects against reproduction of "bad" bacteria, dangerous to health. But did you know that consumption of probiotics can help reduce body weight?

The research carried out at Stanford University in the US have shown that the presence of probiotics is much higher among people who are thinner than those who have problems with excess weight or are chronically obese. That is why they came to the conclusion that increased amounts of probiotics in the body can lead to a reduction in body weight.

What actually happens in the intestine?

Probiotics play a key role when it comes to digesting food. They are supplied with intestinal enzymes that are required for the digestion of the various nutrients, are responsible for synthesizing some vitamins, and increasing the absorption of energy from food.

Probiotics can help in regulation of certain mechanisms that regulate weight. Specifically, the aforementioned research has followed the relationship between the immune system, metabolism, intestinal bacteria, digestion and obesity, and have come to the conclusion that increasing the body weight depends not only on increased food intake, but also on a very sensitive mutual relation of intestinal bacteria and metabolism. Therefore, the good bacteria that are found in the intestine may help in the regulation of metabolism.

Probiotics have beneficial effects not only on the digestive and immune system but also on the overall health of the body. But, did you know how important role probiotic cultures have in reducing the body weight, regulating the endocrine system, reducing the subcutaneous fat - especially in the abdomen, raising energy and the health of soft hollow organs, including the digestive tract, urinary tract and mucous membrane.

Chapter 1: Bacteria and obesity

The Biodesign Institute at the Arizona State University in collaboration with the Mayo Clinic conducted a small research on nine people, which is not enough to be recognized in scientific circles, but definitely showed the direction to be followed in the research. From these nine people, they selected three with normal body weight, three people who were obese and three people who were on the gastric bypass surgery.

The beginning of the study showed that all three groups of people had different types of bacteria in their intestines. But as time passed by, people who undergo gastric bypass surgery had a composition of intestinal bacteria much more like those people who had normal body weight, thanks to proper diet after surgery.

With further understanding of the importance and role of different types of probiotics in our body, there is a possibility that in the future, it will be able to prevent obesity in healthy and proper way, and not only with a lighter body weight reduction, but also by preventing obesity before it happens, and all thanks to the knowledge of the composition of intestinal microflora.

What should you eat?

For the natural development of probiotics in the body, you need to eat fermented foods rich in lactic acid bacteria, and these are bacteria that are responsible for the actual fermentation.

Sour milk and other dairy products:

- yogurt
- kefir
- buttermilk
- yeast
- sour or fresh cabbage
- borscht
- peppermint
- dark chocolate
- ginger tea

Food with prebiotics (food that helps in the development of probiotics)

- bananas
- onions
- garlic
- honey
- artichokes

Of course, varied and healthy diet, rich in fruits and vegetables will help in improving and restoring intestinal flora, which will improve digestion and regulate metabolism, and therefore the thinness.

Chapter 2: Probiotics and reduction in body weight studies

According to a recent study probiotics seem to affect the reduction of body fat, especially in the abdomen. They accomplish this by regulating the hormones that send signals to our brain associated with feelings of hunger, preventing the absorption of fat calories in the intestines and raising our energy level, giving us the motivation to exercise and strength for everyday activities that stimulate our metabolism to digest and burn fat. The results of this study suggest that probiotics prevent the absorption of fat in the intestine and this could be an effective weapon for weight loss.

Pete Jones from the University of Manitoba in Canada claims that normally we digest all groups of food and absorb all the calories. Probiotics affect the absorption of fat calories, so more calories came out and there is less abdominal fat to be filled up.

The study was conducted on a small sample of participants who were slightly overweight, and weight loss effect was fairly modest, so even if the results were confirmed, probiotics would not eliminate the need for maintaining a proper diet and exercise.

Good intestinal bacteria

Probiotics, or active bacterial cultures can change the ecology of the bacteria that are found in human intestines. Beneficial bacteria can improve the condition of depression, calm the stomach problems and even fight sinus infections.

Given that other studies have shown that intestinal bacteria can change the way the body absorbs calories from food, Jones and his colleagues wanted to see if it can influence the weight reduction. Jones' team made of 28 volunteers consumed yogurt daily. In yogurt were added bacteria *Lactobacillus fermentum* or *Lactobacillus amylovorus* to half of the participants. To isolate the effect of the bacteria, researchers have provided all the food that the participants ate during the study.

After a month and a half, those who ate probiotic supplements had between 3% and 4% less body fat than at the beginning of the study. Most of this was the loss of fat in the abdomen, which may be associated with heart diseases. Researchers do not know why the majority of the participants lost abdominal fat.

The team believes that the bacteria reduce body fat because the intestine prevented the body to absorbed calories. The liver secretes soapy chemicals called bile salts, which mix with the fat and help to digest the same. At the same probiotics interfere with destruction of these bile salts and the absorption of fat.

Unlike other diet supplements that prevent the absorption of fat in the intestine, probiotics are not causing unpleasant side effects.

A related study found out that the number of *bifidobacterium* in infants aged between six and eight months was twice as high at children with a healthy body weight compared with children who are overweight, while the level of bacteria *staphylococcus aureus* (otherwise one of the most common causes of infections from injuries) was lower. These results could explain why children fed with breast milk are in reduced risk of obesity, since bifidobacteria survives in the intestines of these children.

Two other studies have showed that obese people have about 20% more bacteria from originating from bacteria called *firmicutes* and nearly 90% less bacteria called *bacteroidetes* than skinny people have.

Firmicutes bacteria help the body to extract calories from complex sugars that store these calories into fat.

When these microbes were transplanted into mice of normal weight, these mice have begun to receive twice as much fat. So this is one of the possible explanations of how microflora in the intestine may play a key role in regulating the body weight. It was found that probiotics can help with the metabolic syndrome that often goes hand in hand with obesity.

Chapter 3: Do you need to lose weight?

The definition of obesity

Obesity is an excessive weight gain due to increased accumulation of body fat and can seriously damage human health. It is closely associated with various diseases such as myocardial infarction and other cardio vascular disease, Type 2 Diabetes, various cancers, problems with bones and joints, and many others.

According to the World Health Organization, the number of obese people in the world has doubled in the last 35 years. It is particularly worrying that the number of obese children is growing rapidly and they all remain obese for the rest of their lives which seriously undermines their health.

Factors that influence the development of obesity

These factors can be hereditary, endocrine disorders, but the most common problems today, in which we include 95% of all, is that obese people practice sedentary lifestyle, lack of physical activity and excessive intake of food rich in carbohydrates. Therefore, the majority of them can be successfully treated with a combination of correctly programmed and dosed physical activity and a proper diet.

Hormones leptin and ghrelin control signals that tell our brain if we are fed or hungry. In a healthy and well-balanced intestinal flora they function normally. However, when the intestinal flora is missing the intestinal bacteria, it is not functioning normally, and we cannot regulate appetite, which often leads to overeating.

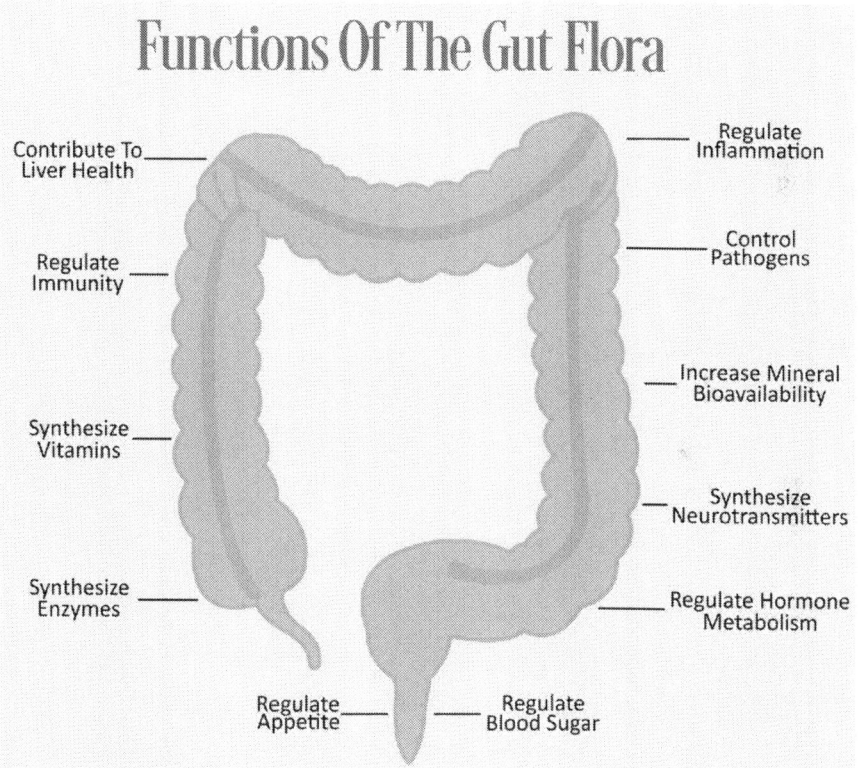

Functions Of The Gut Flora

Contribute To Liver Health

Regulate Immunity

Synthesize Vitamins

Synthesize Enzymes

Regulate Appetite

Regulate Blood Sugar

Regulate Inflammation

Control Pathogens

Increase Mineral Bioavailability

Synthesize Neurotransmitters

Regulate Hormone Metabolism

Probiotics help in establishing a balance in the intestinal flora and thus affect the functionality of the hormone responsible for regulating appetite.

Attendance of probiotics in our system plays a critical role in digestion and energy production. In the absence of friendly bacteria in our system, the efficiency of digestion is reduced, and our body has to use additional amounts of energy to digest food, resulting in a lower level of energy in the body. Decreased energy level is associated with reduced level of motivation for exercise or other activities that would burn the fat and help in reducing weight. Although the intake of probiotic bacteria does not give a lot of energy, their positive activity in the intestines can improve digestion.

Be sure to keep in mind that you take care of quality sources of probiotic bacteria in your diet. Probably the best source is natural fermented food.

Chapter 4: Health benefits of kefir

Kefir is a naturally fermented dairy drink with sour refreshing taste and a light hint of fresh yeast (or very lightly flavored beer), which is made from kefir grains. It is believed that kefir is originating from the Caucasus. It is old more than 1 000 years ago. The inhabitants of the Caucasus are known for their longevity and good health. They live almost without any diseases, which is attributed to their daily and unlimited consumption of kefir. Kefir grains in our regions are often called the *Tibetan mushroom or kefir grains.*

Kefir grains that look like cooked cauliflower are a mixture of proteins, amino acids, lactic acid bacteria, acetic bacteria and yeast strains. Kefir grains live and reproduce in milk and have no shelf life, they can live forever. Numerous attempts of microbiologists to produce kefir granules in a laboratory persistently end up in failure. The question where they come from and how they are formed remains without a scientific answer. Legend says that the kefir grains are a gift from God that God sent the Israelites when Moses led them out of Egypt to the Promised Land.

Kefir has many positive effects in the prevention of a large number of diseases and conditions. Among other things, it is considered that:

- acts as the strongest tool against allergies and food intolerance;
- acts as a natural antibiotic;
- is reducing inflammatory (inflammatory) disease such as rheumatism and arthritis;
- strengthens the immune system and accelerates the healing of the body;
- improves digestion and proper utilization of nutrients from food;
- heals bowel diseases such as IBS (irritable bowel syndrome), intestinal permeability syndrome, constipation, diarrhea, bloating;
- fights against gastric diseases such as gastritis and gastric ulcer;
- cleanses and detoxifies the body;
- improves the function of liver and acts against gallstones;
- helps with cardiovascular disease;
- lowers blood sugar, high blood pressure and high blood fat (triglycerides);
- treats fungal diseases;
- helps to stop the growth of the malignant cells;
- normalizes metabolism and thus promotes loss of excess weight;
- helps with insomnia and depression;

- helps with bronchitis and asthma;
- helps with psoriasis and eczema

Chapter 5: Homemade kefir

Kefir grains can be purchased from someone who has already got himself a real kefir at home. Contact with such a person, it is most easily established over the internet, and granules can be easily packed inside a plastic bag with a little milk and mail. They reproduce quickly, so they can be shared with others.

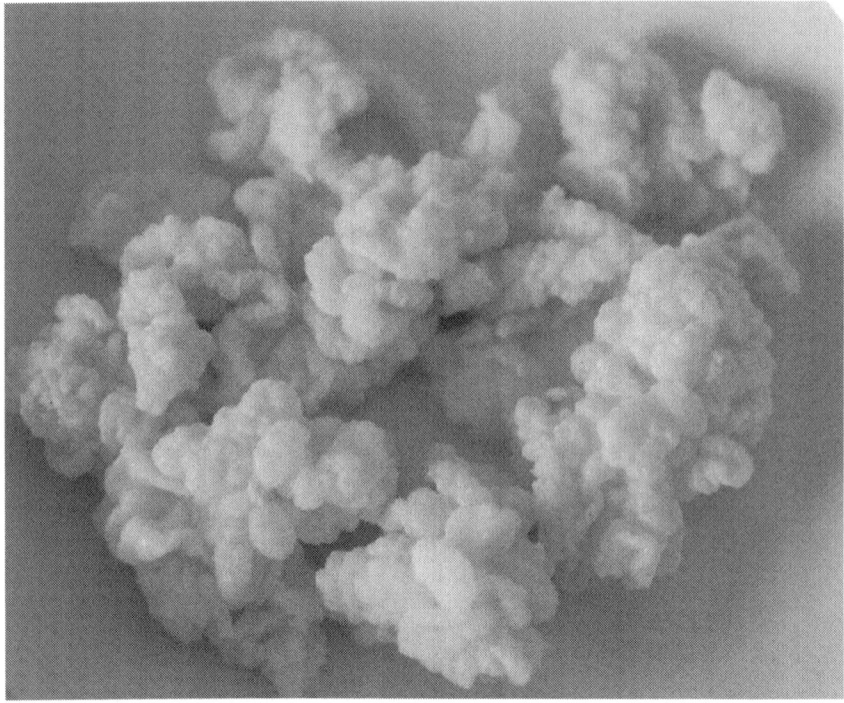

Kefir can be easily prepared at home. Put a small amount of grain and milk in a jar, close the lid and leave at room temperature to ferment for 24 hours. Kefir granules feed with milk sugar and they produce lactic acid and CO_2. After 24 hours, filter kefir through a colander, mixing it with a spoon. Kefir grains that are left put into new milk, a strained kefir is finished and ready to drink. You can drink it right away or cool in the refrigerator.

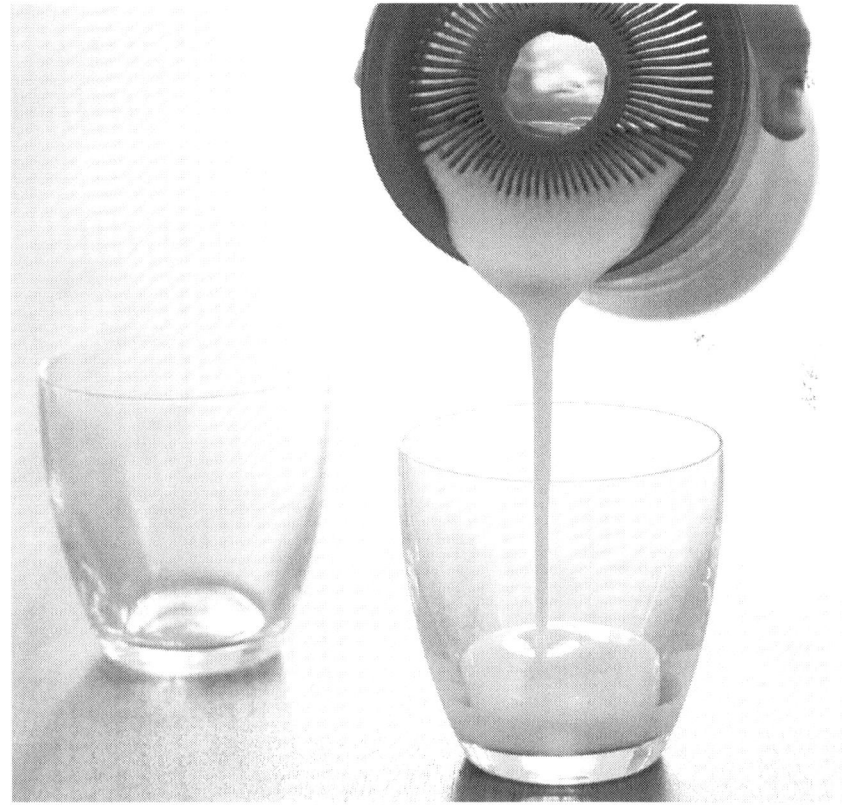

One full tablespoon of granules is enough for about half a liter of kefir. For preparation of kefir it is best to use fresh milk (cow or goat), but in the absence of such, buy milk and it will do the job. Kefir is prepared when milk is fermented, i.e. when thickened and looking like yogurt. At the bottom of the jar may be separated liquid – kefir whey, a beverage that may be thicker, more cream-like or watery, depending on the type of milk and the temperature of fermentation. For preparing kefir you can use wood and stainless steel spoons and strainers, but do not keep it in plastic or metal containers because plastic emits chemicals and a metal reacts with acidic content. It is best stored in glass jars. Distilled grains do not need to be rinsed with water, it's enough to put them into new milk and leave it to ferment all over again. For therapeutic purposes, to improve health, people may consume a liter kefir daily. Well, for starters it is good to start with a smaller dose, for example, deciliter a day, then gradually increase the amount. Kefir is radically changing the composition of the intestinal flora. It successfully destroys pathogenic bacteria and occupies their place, and this can cause transient indigestion in some people. People sensitive to dairy products usually tolerate kefir, because the fermentation process dissolves milk components difficult to digest. The bacteria from kefir break down the milk sugar lactose, so it can be used by people who are lactose intolerant. Minerals from milk, for example calcium, become biologically available from the fermentation process (can be easier to use).

People who pay attention to carbohydrate intake (LCHF diet) may reduce the sugar content of kefir in a way that after straining they leave kefir one to two days at room temperature to "mature". This kefir contains the least possible amount of sugar and the content of vitamin B1, B6 and B9 (folic acid) is increased. Increasing the alcohol content in kefir can range from 0.08% to 2%. The usual amount of alcohol in one-day kefir is 0.08 to 0.1%. Strained kefir which ripens should not be tightly folded, but only covered with the lid, it is a good to mix it twice a day.

If you want to take a break in preparing kefir, maybe go on a trip or something, mix granules with cold water, cover them with a little milk and store in the refrigerator, you can keep them this way for about 7 days. If you want to "save" them for a longer time- washed and dried granules can be frozen or dried. When you want to reactivate granules, put them in a little milk at the room temperature and wait for them to "reload". The first and second day, add a little milk, and discard it after draining. On the third day, kefir can work as usual.

The excess cells that reproduce should be removed periodically. If you do not have someone to give this extra kefir, freeze or eat it. Kefir is not much of an experience for chewing, so mix it with other ingredients in a delicious smoothie.

Chapter 6: Top strategies for beginners to start losing weight: 12 kefir diets

Kefir is a unique, low-calorie product, easily digestible and rich in nutrients. And of course, kefir is a basic factor in many diets aimed at weight loss, but is also present as a secondary food (if you can call it that) in some diets, in combination with apples, buckwheat, etc.

1. "Clean" diet with kefir

It lasts three days and you drink only 1-1.5 liter of kefir without sugar each day, divided into five or six portions at regular intervals. Although you will get hungry, you will lose 3-4 pounds.

2. Kefir diet from the nutritional institute

It lasts 21 days. During these three weeks, you can lose up to 10 pounds. There are no special recipes for breakfast, lunch and dinner, there are especially suitable foods or something that cannot be eaten, but the basic principles are easy to understand.

The most important thing is to reduce calorie intake. It is clear that this means the expulsion of white sugar, bread, potatoes and fried foods from your diet. At least half of fat that you enter into the body must be of plant origin. Meat and fish should be low-fat and milk skimmed (this also refers to dairy products). You can eat fruit and vegetables that do not contain starch in immoderate quantities. Drink a maximum of one liter of liquids per day, and at least a liter of water in which you kept kefir, a half-liter can be replaced with water or natural juice. You can eat up to 5 grams of salt. Divide your food into 5-6 meals a day and eat at equal intervals.

3. Winter diet with kefir

This diet should not be practiced more than three days and do not repeat it without a month apart. How many pounds you will lose depends on your body and health (height, weight, age, etc.).

Breakfast: a cup of coffee with milk, omelet and a cabbage salad; or a cup of tea with honey, a slice of bread with butter, one boiled egg and wheat porridge.

Lunch: baked apple or a cup of kefir cocktails/ smoothies

Afternoon snack: a glass of kefir or apples and a piece of cheese

Before dinner: a beetroot salad, braised carrots, chicken soup, a piece of bread; or soup with mushrooms, meat and cabbage

Dinner: a cup of tea, fish fried in vegetable oil with roasted potatoes

Before bed: a glass of kefir or skimmed milk.

4. Diet with kefir and fruit

During this diet, it is necessary to drink 1.5-2 liters of kefir a day and you can eat fruit in unlimited quantities. This diet can be practiced up to 3-4 consecutive days. Thus, you will lose of 2-3 pounds in three days on average.

5. Post-holiday diet with kefir

This kefir diet is usually practiced after holidays. The first reason is to release the body from the excessive food and the second is not to get used to excessive food intake, which quickly leads to overweight. This diet should be followed one day, avoiding the food that you eat often during the holidays, if you have not gained weight and you only want to recover your body.

Breakfast: a glass of kefir, and possibly a piece of bread

Lunch: a glass of kefir or fruit (preferably apple)

Afternoon snack: two apples and a glass of kefir, or juice

Before dinner: a glass of kefir or fruit

Dinner: piece of cheese and one or two apples

Before bed: a glass of kefir or milk.

6. Skipping diet with kefir

It can be followed as much as you want, because it is not difficult. How much weight you lose depends on your body and its current situation and needs. This diet is very simple. One day you drink only kefir with 1% fat (in abundance), the next day you can eat anything without restrictions. Sometimes, instead of kefir, you can drink plain water. The third day is same as the first, and so on.

7. Diet with kefir and apples

This diet should be followed 9 days, but it has a long term effect. You can lose up to 9 kilos during the diet.

The first three days: drink only 1.5 liters of low-fat kefir

Another three days: eat 1.5 kg of fresh apples

The third three days: drink 1.5 liters of low-fat kefir

From time to time, while following this diet, you may experience nausea, so sometimes you can consume a food rich in carbohydrates and proteins.

8. The nine-day diet with kefir

It's hard to follow; but it is the diet for losing about 9 pounds. You have to return carefully to the old diet regime once the diet is over. Do not overdo immediately with a highly caloric food.

The first three days: kefir with 1% fat in unlimited quantities and 100 grams of boiled rice (no salt)

Another three days: kefir with 1% fat in unlimited quantities, 100 grams of boiled chicken (white meat without salt)

The third three days: kefir with 1% fat in unlimited quantities, fresh apples in unlimited quantities.

9. The eight-day diet with kefir

This diet is difficult considering the quality of food and the amount of food you eat, because the nutritional value of foods is insufficient for daily needs if you want to function normally. Before you start this diet, it is necessary to consult with your doctor. If you have any disease, do not follow this diet.

Arrange all the food in 3-4 meals throughout the day. Do not modify products or add anything (especially sugar or salt). You can drink water in unlimited quantities.

First day: half a liter of kefir, 3-4 boiled potatoes

Second day: half a liter of kefir, a pound of dried fruit

Third day: half a liter of kefir, a pound of cottage cheese

Fourth day: half a liter of kefir, a pound of sour cream

Fifth day: half a liter of kefir, 300 grams of cooked chicken

Sixth day: half a liter of kefir, 2 kg of fresh fruit

Seventh day: 2-3 liters of kefir

Eighth day: mineral water in unlimited quantities

10. The one-week kefir diet

During this diet all foods are prepared without salt and sugar. Since it is difficult, follow it every two or three months, not more often. How much you will lose weight depends on the characteristics and condition of your body, but on average it is about 5 pounds.

Day one: 1.5 l kefir and 5 boiled potatoes

Second day: 1.5 l of kefir and 100 grams of cooked chicken (preferably white meat)

Third day: 1.5 l of kefir and 100 grams of boiled meat (preferably beef)

Fourth day: 1.5 l of kefir and 100 grams of cooked fish

Fifth day: 1.5 l of kefir and fruit and vegetables (bananas and grapes are not permitted, because they are too caloric)

Sixth day: 1.5-2 liters of kefir

Seventh day: mineral water in unlimited quantities

It is best to drink one glass of kefir every 3-4 hours. In addition, during the day, you can change the type of kefir you drink. For example, drink low fat kefir, followed by food, than drink greasier kefir. It is better to drink mineral water than usual. During this diet you should not drink coffee or tea.

11. The five-day kefir diet

During this diet you can lose up to 5 pounds. A feature of this diet is that diet must be adhered strictly by hour:

7:00 cup of tea without sugar

9:00 salad made of grated carrots (two medium) seasoned with vegetable oil

11:00 200 grams of boiled meat, veal or chicken (white meat)

13:00 an apple

15:00 hard-boiled egg

17:00 an apple

19:00 10 prunes

21:00 glass of kefir

12. Fasting days with kefir and whey

When you want to cleanse the body, follow this diet for a few days. The effect is based on the fact that kefir and fresh cheese regulate metabolism, body normally consumes energy and thus comes to weight loss. Those days when you drink whey, eat 500-600 grams of low-fat cottage cheese, divided into 5-6 meals; you can drink only water. The day when you drink only kefir, divide 1.5 l of kefir into 5-6 servings. On the day when you combine whey and kefir, consume 250-300 grams of nonfat cottage cheese and 750 ml of kefir also divided in 5-6 meals.

Chapter 7: Weight loss for obese people

There are two ways to lose weight for obese people with the help of kefir. The first one is losing weight on a longer period of time, with the help of kefir diet. This way you will lose 4-6 kilograms per month. This diet is for less obese people who want to normalize their weight.

The second diet is for obese people, and for 2 months you can lose up to 25 kg of excessive weight. Neither one is harmful to health. You can use them depending on your degree of obesity.

Regular diet program:

To lose weight, you need to drink 100 ml of kefir every day, half an hour after each meal. Once or twice a week is useful to make a restrictive day based on kefir – drink 1-1.5 l of kefir throughout the day. If *the kefir day* is too strenuous for you, try to implement restrictive day with the help of apples and pears.

The fasting day menu:

The first breakfast (9:00 to 9:30): Apple (raw or roasted) and a glass of kefir

The second breakfast (10:00 to 11:30): pear, apple and a glass of kefir

Lunch (13:00 to 14:00): a glass of kefir and a piece of black bread

Dinner (17:00 to 17:30): a salad made of pears and apples (or grated apples and carrots), topped with kefir.

One hour before bedtime drink a glass of kefir with a teaspoon of honey.

In order to lose weight in this way, kefir should be consumed 20 days. Then you make a 10 days pause, and then continue with the diet. This diet can be followed entire year, or until the desired weight.

The value of this diet is reduction of 4-6 kilograms per month. It is sustainable and stable weight loss. In addition, it normalizes the intestinal microflora, eliminates cholesterol; hormones and metabolism are returning to normal. The result is complete normalization of body weight. Nutritionists say it's easy to lose weight, if you limit the intake of sweet, fatty foods and products made from white flour in addition to consuming kefir.

Diet program for obese:

Treatment of obesity with the help of kefir consists in certain rules:

One week you are on a regular diet. The next week you are following the diet program and so on.

Before you start to follow the diet program, follow a restrictive day (as described above). After the first week of the diet program, return to a regular diet for a week. Limit the intake of sweets, fatty and starchy foods. Then, you continue to repeat the diet scenario: the next week should follow the diet program, then regular program and so on.

During a regular diet, adhere to schedule to consuming meals by hours. Spread your food in 6 meals in the same time period until 6 p.m. After 6 p.m. - do not eat.

When having a hunger pang you can drink an additional 100 ml of kefir.

Dietary restrictions: you should restrict the fluid intake during the diet week- do not drink more than 0.5 liters of water, except for the fifth day when you should drink 1.5 liters of mineral water.

Food is divided into four parts, and kefir in 5 portions. The last portion of kefir should be consumed an hour before bedtime.

Day 1: 400 grams of boiled potatoes without salt and 0.5 liter of kefir

Day 2: 400 grams of low-fat cheese and 0,5l of kefir

Day 3: 400 g of fruit (except bananas and grapes) and 0.5 liters kefir

Day 4: 400 grams of boiled chicken breast without salt and 0.5 liters of kefir

Day 5: 400 grams of fruit and 0,5l of kefir

Day 6: 1.5 liters of non-carbonated mineral water

7 day: 400 grams of fruit and 400 ml of kefir

Scientific research on a group of volunteers showed reduction of body weight for about 8-10 kg for 2 weeks, on the average- 25 kg in 2 months.

What you need to know before you start following the diet with kefir for the first time:

Begin to consume kefir 100 ml per day, gradually increasing the dose until the body adjusts to it. In the first 10-14 days of consuming kefir, the activity of the intestines increases. It manifests in the form of increased emissions of gases, frequent discharge and discoloration of urine. But it is a normal reaction, a sign that the process of cleaning and detoxification of the body has begun.

After ten days, the reaction of the organism stops and it comes to the improvement of the general situation. Pregnant women and people with intolerance to dairy products should not drink kefir. People with increased acid should pay attention.

If you consume drugs, practice a pause between taking drugs and kefir for 3 hours. During the consumption of kefir you should abstain from alcohol.

Chapter 8: The best recipes for a healthy intestinal flora

After you have found out how much probiotics and prebiotics in food are important for a healthy intestinal flora, the next step is to prepare some great recipes. In this situation we have prepared 3 outstanding recipes.

Light cream soup

Ingredients:

- 2 small leeks cut into rings
- 2 medium onions diced
- 2 large potatoes peeled and cut into cubes
- 3 cloves of finely chopped garlic
- 4 cups of vegetable broth
- 2 teaspoons fresh of rosemary leaves
- 1 tablespoon of olive oil
- salt and pepper

Preparation:

Heat the olive oil at the medium heat, and add the leeks and onions. Season is with salt and sauté for five minutes, then add the garlic and sauté another minute. Add potatoes and vegetable broth, cover, lower the temperature and cook for 20 minutes. Leave it to cool a bit and mix with the rosemary leaves. Pour the soup back into the pot, heat to the boiling point and remove from the stove. Serve warm.

A phenomenal leek salad:

Ingredients:

- 4 medium beets
- 4 small leeks cut into pieces
- A bunch of finely chopped parsley

For the dressing:

- 1 cup of finely chopped walnuts
- 2 cloves of finely chopped garlic
- 1/4 teaspoon of hot peppers
- 1/4 cup of apple cider vinegar
- 2 teaspoons of balsamic vinegar
- 1 teaspoon of sesame oil
- 3 tablespoons of olive oil
- salt and pepper to taste

Preparation:

Mix all the ingredients for the dressing and leave them on a side. Cook the beets and strain them. Leave them to cool, peel and cut into cubes. Cook leeks in salted water for about ten minutes and then strain it. Rinse leeks under cold water, cut into pieces and pour into a salad bowl along with beets. Pour the dressing, gently stir and sprinkle with chopped parsley.

Salad with radishes and onions:

Prebiotics in food are extremely important for the entire immune system, so we have prepared for you another great recipe.

Ingredients:

- 2 bunches of radish
- 200 g of spinach
- 1 large carrot
- 1/2 of lettuce
- red onion
- 8 cherry tomatoes
- parmesan
- 3 tablespoons of olive oil
- 2 tablespoons of lemon juice
- salt and pepper, to taste

For the dressing:

- 2 dl of sour cream
- tablespoon of olive oil
- tablespoon of lemon juice

- parsley
- salt and pepper, to taste

Preparation:

Wash the vegetables first, then clean and chop. Tear pieces of lettuce leaves and put into salad. Add the leaves of spinach and other vegetables. Season it with salt and pepper. Add two tablespoons of olive oil and lemon juice, and stir well. In particular, mix sour cream with lemon juice and olive oil, season with salt and pepper and add the chopped parsley. Pour over the salad and sprinkle with the sliced parmesan cheese.

Chapter 9: Fast weight loss is dangerous for your body

Dieting without exercise is very bad for health! It turned out that starvation brings more harm than good. It turns out that you can have much more weight than the regular, and be quite healthy assuming that you are physically active.

Following the restrictive diet is not a good way to lose weight. It has been shown that even 95% of people who have been on a diet regain their lost weight within three or five years with a higher percentage of body fat.

Restrictive diets drastically restrict calorie intake, which slows down the metabolism, leading to depressive states, facilitating the loss of muscle mass rather than fat mass, which leads to becoming thinner with very poor body composition.

Starvation mode does not encourage long lasting changes in lifestyle, but only temporary, and leads to termination of diet habits and quick return to old eating habits. Thus, fast return of the old weight IS INEVITABLE.

Exercise will not only remove the fat from specific areas, but will program the proportion of waste depending on genetics, gender and hormonal levels. By increasing the volume of muscles in certain areas of the body, you can change the shape of the body, plus increase a specific loss of fat, because the more muscles you have- the more fat you burn!

Bringing the condition of the body and the whole body in good shape is certainly not an easy job. Increased physical activity and controlled diet are natural and healthy way to do it, but it is also required to have a strong and unbreakable spirit, support and supervision in order to avoid the negative consequences of their use.

Chapter 10: You need to feel comfortable while losing weight

Certainly, the best way to achieve the desired, permanent and healthy weight is properly dosed physical exercise and correct eating habits. To be successful in this, you must have a high level of motivation and ability to change your lifestyle.

However, a set of basic rules should be followed in order to succeed in achieving your objectives:

- Establish the energy balance, i.e. the number of calories consumed should be less than the number of calories spent;
- The gradual reduction in calories, because sudden reduction can slow metabolism, slow down the function of the thyroid gland and lead to a decrease in muscle mass rather than fat mass. Daily caloric needs for women is about 2000 calories; for men is 2500, but still, this depends on weight, height, age, body composition, daily activities. From the standpoint of good health, reducing the daily intake below 1200 calories for women and 1800 for men is not good.
- For 1kg of fat loss per week it is required to achieve a negative energy balance of more than 7000 calories;

- Throw out simple sugars and trans fats from the diet;
- The efficiency loss of fat requires greater physical activity and it must be included during most days during the week. It must be adapted to your age, health status and the current physical condition;
- Training length varies from 45 minutes up to 90 minutes;
- Many studies have shown that combination of aerobic and anaerobic activities are much more effective than just aerobic (walking, running, swimming, biking ...) or just anaerobic (weightlifting, for example...). Aerobic activities accelerate the metabolism of fats which are consumed during training, while highly intense anaerobic exercise posture metabolism at a high level for hours after training (3 to 14 hours, depending on the intensity). The body metabolizes fat 9 times more for each calorie consumed during anaerobic compared to aerobic activity. Anaerobic activity in highly obese is difficult to perform at the beginning of the process, it is necessary to gradually introduce them as it can cause serious injury and other side effects;
- Regular and good sleep - at least 7 to 8 hours a day is A MUST, and it is very important not to lose control over the food intake
- Losing weight through sweating in the sauna or steam bath is current only at the expense of lost fluids. As

soon as the water regains, body weight returns to its old weight

Increased physical activity leads to increase in muscle mass, decrease of fat body mass and smaller scale of the body, while your weight can remain the same. If your weight loss doesn't go as planned, you need an additional motivation for increasing the volume of training and further correction of nutrition.

A higher percentage of muscle means results in higher energy consumption. 1kg of muscle can burn between 50 and 100 calories per day, while 1 kg of fat burns only 3 calories.

Negative energy balance will cause to consume fat for energy and compensate for the calorie deficiency.

In addition to improving the quality of your life, exercise brings health to your body. Here are some positive effects of exercise:

- Relieve stress, because it burns many chemical substances that are harmful to the body,
- The muscles are relaxed after exercise
- Is a natural antidepressant
- Increases the production of good cholesterol, which regulates fatty deposits in the arteries, thus preventing the formation of blood vessel diseases
- Reduces overweight
- Improves metabolism

- It strengthens the heart muscle and improves its performance
- Improves blood system, thus the ability to get oxygen and nutrients to better distribute them in the body
- Improves the performance and capacity of the lungs, thus the introduction of oxygen in the body.

Conclusion

Thank you again for purchasing this book!

We've discovered that probiotics effectively regulate our body weight and intestinal flora.

Our organism has billions of bacteria, so our body can be thought of as a huge living area, while the bacteria are our tenants. Many of them only live in our digestive organs. At the same time, each person has his own unique bacterial flora, such as fingerprints, which are different for each of us. Some scientific directions even suggest that the bacteria we carry in ourselves have a similar role as some human organs and they are, by relevance, comparable to the liver. Thus, the bacterial microflora of man is to be nurtured in the proper way and maintained normal.

Good bacteria help us to digest food, and actively participate in absorption of nutrients. If there aren't good bacteria, we would not actually be able to digest everything that we are normally accustomed to eat. Not only that, these days it is considered that the highest authority of the immune system in humans have human intestine. The use of certain drugs, bad diet, elevated body temperature, and stress can lead to disorders of the intestinal microflora. As a result, there are all sorts of health problems, from stomach bloating and diarrhea to blemished immunity. The presence of good bacteria in the intestine, not only protects the intestinal mucosa, but also prevents the uncontrolled multiplication of harmful bacteria. When the good bacteria in our stomach are sufficient in number, there is less space for bad bacteria and other pathogenic microorganisms (fungi, viruses ...).

Probiotics are good bacteria (live cultures of microorganisms) that have a positive impact on the microflora of our digestive system. Given the importance of these friendly bacteria, it is important to keep yourself healthy bacterial environment.

Recent studies have recognized the differences in bacteria of the digestive system in people with normal weight and those with overweight. Scientists believe that the differences in the composition of bacteria potentially contribute to the development of obesity. Many studies have proved that consuming probiotics can contribute to weight reduction and regulating the composition of bacteria in the digestive tract.

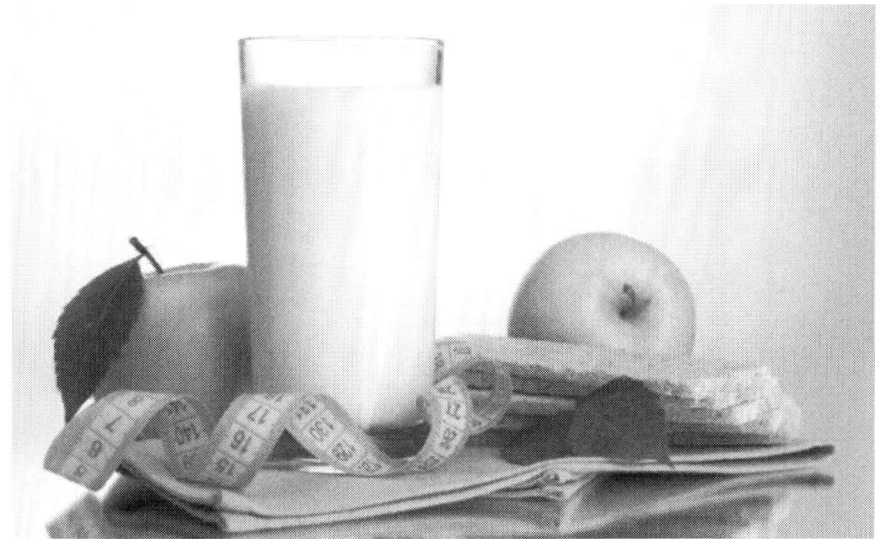

Finally, if you enjoyed this book, then I'd like to ask you for a favor, would you be kind enough to leave a review for this book on Amazon? It'd be greatly appreciated!

Thank You and Good Luck!

Printed in Great Britain
by Amazon